HEALTHY SMOOTHIES, BOWLS & TREATS

EASY DELICIOUS NUTRITION RECIPES WITH SUPERFOODS

EMMA WILLSON

DISCLAIMER

The information provided in this cookbook is intended for general informational purposes only. The recipes, nutritional details, and any health-related information included are not intended to replace professional advice from a qualified healthcare or nutrition professional.

While every effort has been made to ensure the accuracy and completeness of the information presented, individual circumstances and health conditions may vary, and it is crucial to consult with a healthcare professional or a registered dietitian before making significant changes to your diet or lifestyle.

The cookbook's author, publisher, and contributors are not responsible for any adverse effects or consequences resulting from using the information presented herein. Any reliance you place on the information within this cookbook is very much at your own risk.

Allergy and dietary information is based on commonly available information and may not cover all possible allergies or dietary restrictions. The reader must check all ingredients, consider their nutritional needs, and take appropriate precautions.

Recipes and nutritional values in this cookbook may be estimated and vary based on ingredient brands, variations, and portion sizes. Readers should use their discretion and judgment when preparing and consuming the dishes.

By using this cookbook, you agree to absolve the author, publisher, and contributors from any liability, directly or indirectly, arising from using or applying any information presented herein. Always seek professional advice regarding any specific health or dietary concerns.

Please note that this disclaimer does not cover all potential situations or circumstances, and users should use their discretion and consult appropriate professionals as needed.

TABLE OF CONTENTS

TABLE OF CONTENTS

INTRODUCTION

Welcome to "Healthy Smoothies, Bowls, and Treats: Easy and Delicious Superfood Nutrition Recipes." This cookbook is your gateway to a world of delicious and nutritious smoothies that will delight your taste buds and improve your well-being. Each recipe contains tasty fillers and healthy superfoods that are excellent sources of vitamins and minerals. Did you know that adding just one teaspoon of one of these unique gifts of nature gives your body a daily dose of all the essential nutrients? Whether you are a seasoned health enthusiast or just embarking on a wellness journey, this book is your indispensable resource for preparing a variety of delicious and healthy dishes that will be a great addition to main meals or a complete replacement for breakfasts and snacks.

Finding time to prepare delicious and nutritious meals can be difficult in today's fast-paced world. That's where this cookbook comes in handy. We've assembled a collection of easy-to-make recipes full of superfoods - natural energy sources packed with vitamins, minerals, and antioxidants that can help improve your health. These recipes are designed to fit easily into your busy life and make healthy eating easy. Plus, each dish is like a work of art. The variety of flavors and colors will lift your mood and decorate your table.

On these pages, you will find various recipes for every taste. We've got you covered, from invigorating morning smoothies to refreshing and hearty plates and tasty treats that won't interfere with your health goals. Moreover, each recipe is accompanied by stunning full-color pictures that inspire and guide you through preparation.

Whether you want to start your day with a vibrant green smoothie, energize after a workout with a protein bowl, or satisfy your sweet tooth without the guilt, you'll find something here to suit your tastes. With readily available ingredients and easy-to-follow instructions, you'll be whipping up these delicious creations in no time.

But this book is more than just a collection of recipes; it's a path to a healthier, happier you. As you embark on this culinary journey, you'll insatiate your body and deepen your understanding of superfoods' incredible benefits. You'll discover how easy it is to incorporate these nutrient-rich ingredients into your daily diet, helping you achieve and maintain optimal wellness.

So, whether you're a seasoned chef or new to the kitchen, Healthy Smoothies, Bowls & Treats invites you to explore the world of superfoods and get on the delicious path to better health. Get ready to savor the taste of wellness and live a lifestyle that celebrates your taste buds and vitality.

Superfoods are nature's nutritional treasures, offering a cornucopia of health benefits that can revolutionize your well-being. In this chapter, we embark on a journey through a selection of extraordinary superfoods, each with unique attributes contributing to overall health and vitality. Let's delve deeper into the superpowers of each one:

Chia Seeds: Chia seeds are unassuming in size but colossal in nutritional value. Bursting with omega-3 fatty acids, fiber, and antioxidants, they are a powerhouse for promoting heart health, aiding digestion, and providing a sustained energy source. Chia seeds absorb liquids and swell, making them a fantastic ingredient for satisfying thick-textured smoothie bowls. Chia seeds are also a good calcium, potassium, and copper source. Buy chia seeds in their whole seed form, not ground.

Unsweetened Coconut Flakes: Coconut flakes, when unsweetened, offer a bounty of benefits. They are a source of healthy fats that provide sustained energy and promote brain function. Rich in dietary fiber, they also support digestive health and help maintain a feeling of fullness, making them a delightful addition to smoothie bowls or garnish. Coconut also contains omega-3 fatty acids, fiber, phosphorus, and iron.

Turmeric: The golden spice turmeric owes its vibrancy to curcumin, a potent anti-inflammatory compound. Beyond its striking color, turmeric's natural charm lies in its ability to reduce inflammation, support joint health, and bolster the immune system. It imparts an earthy warmth to recipes and pairs wonderfully with fruits, making it an exciting superfood to incorporate into your smoothie concoctions. This incredible spice fights cancer, eases arthritis, and lowers the risk of heart attacks.

Maca: Hailing from the high Andes of Peru, maca root is an adaptogen renowned for its stress-fighting properties. Beyond stress resilience, maca enhances energy levels, boosts mood, and supports hormonal balance. It's an intriguing ingredient to elevate your smoothies, lending them a malty, nutty flavor. This powerful compound contains eight essential amino acids, fatty acids, calcium, magnesium, iron, and potassium. It is also a great hormone-balancing substance. When buying maca powder, always choose organic maca roots.

Cacao: Cacao, the pure form of chocolate, is a treat for the taste buds and a gift to your health. Abounding in antioxidants, magnesium, and mood-enhancing compounds, it promotes heart health, sharpens cognitive function, and provides a guilt-free indulgence. Dark chocolate lovers will relish the addition of raw cacao to their smoothies and bowls. This superfood is rich in flavonoids and decreases LDL.

Ginger Root: Ginger is a time-honored remedy for digestive discomfort and nausea. Its natural anti-inflammatory properties make it a sought-after ingredient for alleviating muscle pain and reducing the risk of chronic diseases. A touch of ginger root can impart a delightful zing to your smoothies and add depth to their flavors. This powerful anti-inflammatory root helps regulate blood sugar and relieve gastrointestinal distress. You can buy this in pure root form, peel it, and add it to smoothies, or buy it in organic powdered form.

Moringa: Moringa leaves, often called the "drumstick tree," are a nutritional treasure trove. Packed with vitamins, minerals, and antioxidants, they bolster the immune system, promote radiant skin, and may even assist in managing blood sugar levels.

The mild, earthy flavor of moringa makes it an easy addition to any superfood recipe.

This nutrient powerhouse contains twenty-five times more iron than spinach and is an excellent source of zinc and magnesium.

Camu Camu: This exotic Amazonian fruit boasts one of the highest vitamin C concentrations of any known food. As a champion of the immune system, camu camu is your ally against illness. Its tangy, tart flavor lends a unique and zesty twist to your smoothie creations. One teaspoon provides 118 percent of the daily recommended intake.

Mangosteen: The "queen of fruits," mangosteen harbors an abundance of antioxidants known as xanthones. These compounds can combat inflammation, slow aging, and defend against various diseases. Incorporating mangosteen into your recipes introduces sweet-tart flavor and health-boosting potential. This superfood is low in calories and has a good vitamin C, magnesium, and potassium serving. It also contains primary cancer-fighting agents.

Matcha: Matcha, a finely ground green tea powder, is a concentrated source of antioxidants, mainly catechins. It's renowned for its metabolism-boosting effects, focus enhancement, and calm alertness. The vibrant green hue of matcha adds an inviting visual appeal to your creations. This tea is full of catechins, an antioxidant shown to help fight and possibly prevent cancer.

Cayenne: Cayenne pepper contains capsaicin, a spicy compound known for its metabolism-boosting prowess. Beyond that, cayenne can alleviate pain, improve circulation, and even aid in weight loss. Its fiery kick can lend a stimulating edge to your smoothies and bowls. This spice is rich in potassium, manganese, flavonoids, and vitamins C, B6, and E. Cayenne has been shown to ease an upset stomach, ulcers, sore throats, coughs, and diarrhea. It is also a great digestive aid.

Almonds: Almonds are a beloved source of nutrition, loaded with healthy fats, fiber, and essential vitamins. They champion heart health, assist in weight management, and provide a steady energy source. This nut has natural calming properties and is rich in stress-reducing vitamins and minerals like magnesium, zinc, and vitamin E. Always purchase organic raw almonds for this book's smoothie and bowl recipes.

Cardamom: This aromatic spice is a flavor enhancer and a health booster. Cardamom aids digestion, reduces inflammation, and may help regulate blood pressure and circulation. Its warm, citrusy notes bring a touch of exotic elegance to your dishes. This spice is an excellent source of potassium, calcium, and magnesium. It contains volatile oils, such as pinene, sabinene, myrcene, phellandrene, and limonene, all aiding digestion, making this spice an excellent addition to your smoothies, smoothie bowls, and baked goods.

Baobab: The fruit of the iconic baobab tree is a nutritional powerhouse, boasting extraordinarily high vitamin C content, fiber, and antioxidants. It reinforces the immune system, supports digestive health and contributes to radiant skin. Baobab's tangy, citrusy flavor makes it a delightful recipe addition. This antioxidant-rich superfood is very high in vitamin C,
which helps produce collagen and elastin. Calcium, copper, iron, magnesium, and potassium are all contained in baobab.

Pumpkin Seeds: Pumpkin seeds, also known as pepitas, are a treasure trove of nutrients, including protein, magnesium, and zinc. They bolster heart health, improve sleep quality, and enhance immune function. Their crunchiness and nutty flavor make them an appealing garnish for bowls and treats.

Spirulina: Spirulina is a blue-green algae celebrated for its dense nutritional profile. It's a powerhouse of protein, iron, and various vitamins. Incorporating spirulina into your recipes can boost energy levels, support immune function, and provide an earthy, algae-like note to your creations.

Acai Powder: Acai berries are renowned for their rich antioxidant content, and acai powder is a convenient way to harness their benefits. It can help improve skin health, promote heart health, and add a berry-like flavor and deep purple color to your dishes.

Goji Berries: Goji berries are small but mighty, packing a punch of vitamins, minerals, and antioxidants. They can boost eye health, enhance immune function, and provide culinary creations with a sweet-tart flavor and chewy texture.

As we delve deeper into this cookbook, you'll discover that these superfoods aren't just ingredients but vital contributors to our recipes' rich tapestry of flavors and health benefits. By incorporating them into your daily diet, you will take a significant step towards a healthier and more energetic lifestyle. So, let's roll up our sleeves and explore the many ways we can harness the potential of these superfoods to create delicious, nutrient-rich culinary.

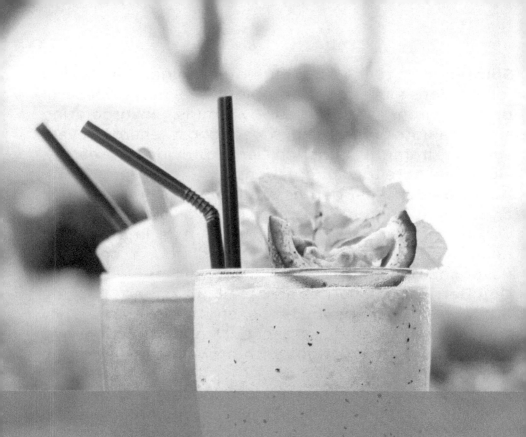

SMOOTHIE

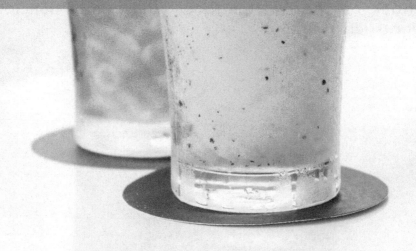

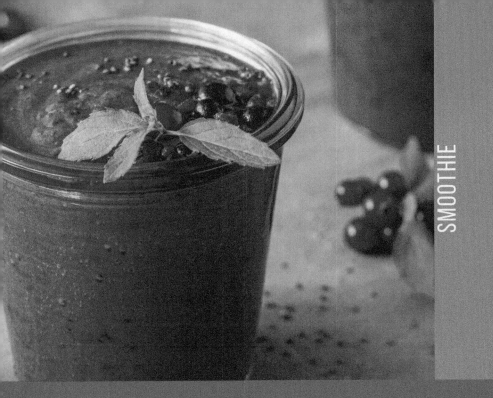

ACAI BERRY AND CHIA SEED SMOOTHIE

INGREDIENTS

- 7 oz acai puree
- 2 tablespoons chia seeds
- 2 cups almond milk
- 1 banana
- 1 cup mixed berries (blueberries, strawberries, raspberries)
- 2 tablespoons honey (adjust to taste)
- Ice cubes (optional for a colder smoothie)

DIRECTIONS

Blend acai puree for the fruity base. Add chia seeds for nutrition. Pour almond milk for the desired consistency. Include a ripe banana for sweetness. Mix in mixed berries for vibrancy. Blend to a vibrant purple. Adjust honey to taste. Pour into glasses when satisfied. Enjoy your Acai Berry and Chia Seed Smoothie!

NUTRITIONAL INFORMATION

(Calories: 290 | Protein: 6g | Carbs: 49g | Fat: 9g

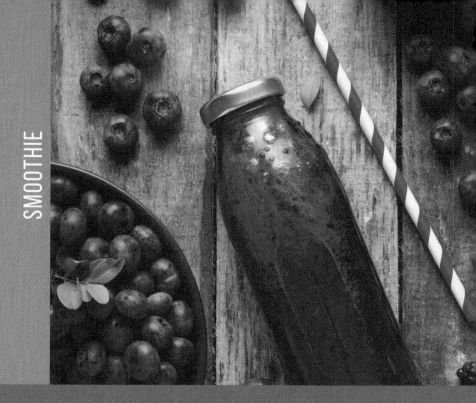

BLACKBERRY ENERGIZING SMOOTHIE

INGREDIENTS

- 7 oz guava puree
- 2 cups fresh blackberries
- 2 cups coconut water
- 1 ripe banana
- 1/4 cup fresh mint leaves
- 1 tablespoon moringa powder

DIRECTIONS

Add the ingredients in the order listed to a high-powered blender. Puree until thick and creamy. Garnish with extra berries and mint sprig if desired, and serve immediately. Blend all the ingredients until you achieve a smooth and velvety texture

NUTRITIONAL INFORMATION

Calories: 280 | Protein: 3g | Carbs: 70g | Fat: 2g

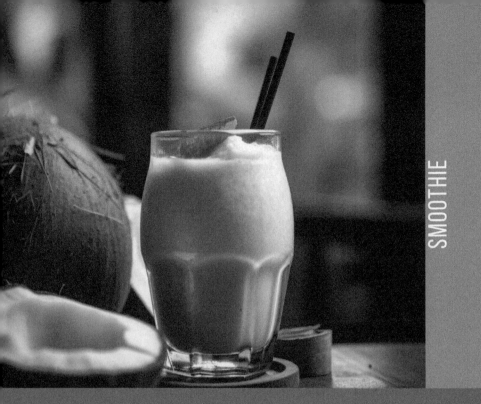

COCONUT DELIGHT SMOOTHIE

INGREDIENTS

- 7 oz mango puree
- 10 fresh figs
- 1 cup coconut milk
- 1 cup coconut water
- 1/4 cup coconut flakes
- Honey (to taste)
- Ice cubes (optional for a colder smoothie

DIRECTIONS

Add the ingredients in the order listed to a high-powered blender. Puree until thick and creamy. Blend all the ingredients until you achieve a smooth and velvety texture. Garnish with coconut flakes, and serve immediately.

NUTRITIONAL INFORMATION

Calories: 350 | Protein: 4g | Carbs: 50g | Fat: 18g

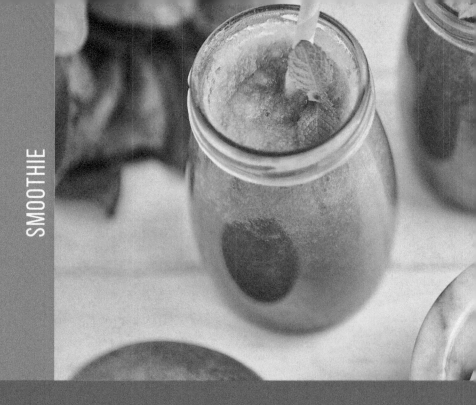

SMOOTHIE

VITAMIN BOOST

INGREDIENTS

- 7 oz apple puree
- 4 Medjool dates, pitted
- 1/2 cup almond milk
- 1 cup orange juice
- 1 cup mango chunks
- 1 cup baby spinach
- 1 tablespoon camu camu powder

DIRECTIONS

Add the ingredients in the order listed to a high-powered blender. Puree until thick and creamy. Blend all the ingredients until you achieve a smooth and velvety texture. Garnish with mint sprig if desired, and serve immediately.

NUTRITIONAL INFORMATION

Calories: 270 | Protein: 4g | Carbs: 65g | Fat: 2g

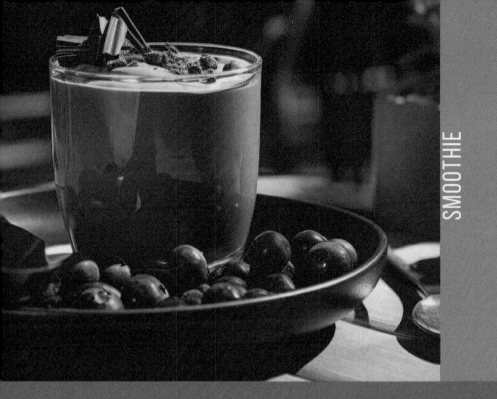

CHEERFUL MORNING

INGREDIENTS

- 1 cup mixed berries
- 2 bananas
- 1 1/2 cups cold-brewed coffee
- 1 cup chocolate almond milk
- 2 tablespoons peanut butter
- 2 tablespoons dark cacao powder

DIRECTIONS

Add the ingredients in the order listed to a high-powered blender. Puree until thick and creamy. Garnish with extra berries and cacao powder, and serve immediately.

NUTRITIONAL INFORMATION

Calories: 250 | Protein: 5g | Carbs: 50g | Fat: 8g |

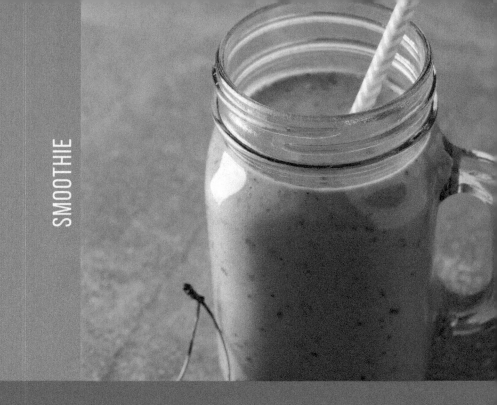

CHERRY TURMERIC SUPERBOOST

INGREDIENTS

- 1 banana
- 2 scoops Supergreens powder
- 1 cup black cherry juice
- 1 cup cherries (frozen or fresh)
- Juice of 1/2 lime
- 1 teaspoon turmeric
- 1/4 teaspoon black pepper

DIRECTIONS

Add the ingredients in the order listed to a high-powered blender. Puree until thick and creamy.

NUTRITIONAL INFORMATION

Calories: 250 | Protein: 3g | Carbs: 56g | Fat: 2g

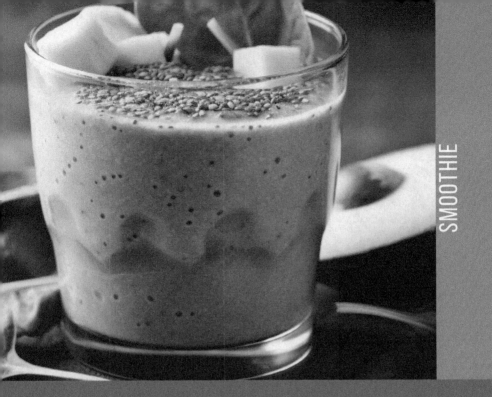

GREEN ENERGY

INGREDIENTS

- 3.5 oz guava puree
- 1 cup baby spinach
- 1 banana
- 1/2 avocado
- 1/4 cup almond butter
- 1 and 1/2 cups almond milk
- Honey (to taste)
- Ice cubes (optional for a colder smoothie)

DIRECTIONS

Add the ingredients in the order listed to a high-powered blender. Blend all the ingredients until you achieve a smooth and velvety texture. Garnish with seeds and spinach. Enjoy!

NUTRITIONAL INFORMATION

Calories: 380 | Protein: 7g | Carbs: 33g | Fat: 26g

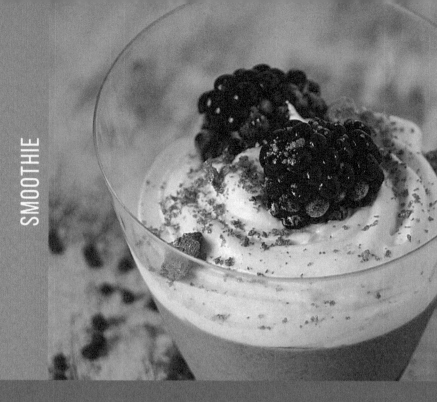

SMOOTHIE

ACAI BERRY CHOCOLATE BLISS

INGREDIENTS

- 7 oz acai puree
- 1 cup blackberries
- 1 banana
- 2 tablespoons cacao powder
- 1 tablespoon maca powder
- 1 tablespoon coconut butter
- Honey (to taste)

DIRECTIONS

Add all ingredients to a high-powered blender. Blend until thick and creamy. Garnish with the cacao nibs and hazelnuts with a few springs of mint and frozen yogurt. Enjoy!

NUTRITIONAL INFORMATION

Calories: 290 | Protein: 3g | Carbs: 44g | Fat: 12g

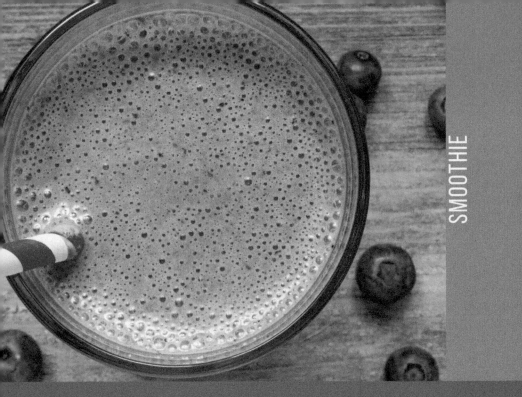

BLUEBERRY BLISS PROTEIN SMOOTHIE

INGREDIENTS

- 3 cups blueberries
- 1 scoop vanilla-flavored pea protein powder
- 1 banana
- 1/2 cup cashew milk
- 1 and 1/2 cups coconut yogurt
- Honey (to taste)
- Ice cubes (optional for a colder smoothie)

DIRECTIONS

Add all ingredients and blender together. Incorporate 1 scoop of vanilla-flavored pea protein powder for a plant-based protein boost. Blend all the ingredients until you achieve a smooth and velvety texture. Serve your smoothie immediately and enjoy the nourishing combination of blueberries, pea protein, and more.

NUTRITIONAL INFORMATION

Calories: 280 | Protein: 8g | Carbs: 45g | Fat: 7g

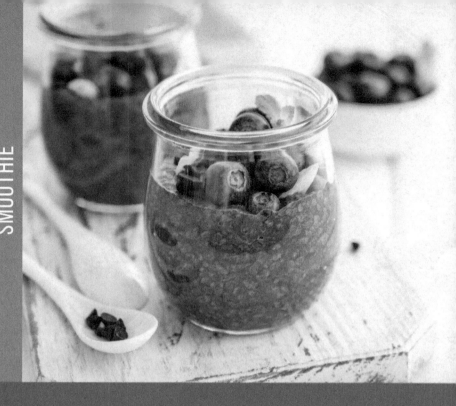

CHOCOLATE DELIGHT SMOOTHIE

INGREDIENTS

- 1 mango
- 1 banana
- 2 tablespoons cacao powder
- 1 cup almond milk
- 1/2 cup blueberries
- Honey (to taste)

DIRECTIONS

Add the ingredients in the order listed to a high-powered blender. Puree until thick and creamy. Garnish with extra berries and mint sprig if desired, and serve immediately. Enjoy!

NUTRITIONAL INFORMATION

Calories: 280 | Protein: 4g | Carbs: 50g | Fat: 8g

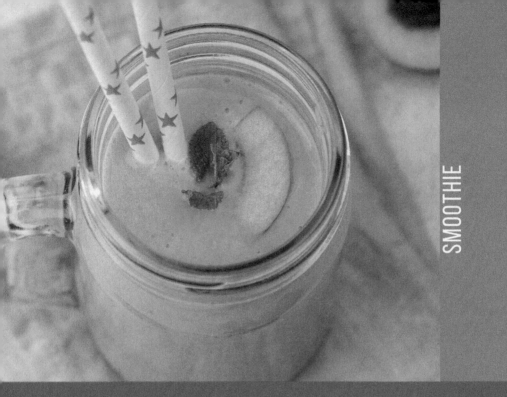

COCONUT PARADISE SMOOTHIE

INGREDIENTS

- 7 oz apricot puree or 6-7 raw apricots
- 2 bananas
- 3 cups coconut water
- 1 cup coconut yogurt
- 2 tablespoons toasted coconut flakes

DIRECTIONS

Add the ingredients in the order listed to a high-powered blender. Puree until thick and creamy. Add more coconut water or flakes to taste your smoothie and adjust the sweetness or thickness. Once your Coconut Paradise Smoothie reaches your preferred texture and flavor, pour it into glasses.

NUTRITIONAL INFORMATION

Calories: 350 | Protein: 4g | Carbs: 70g | Fat: 9g

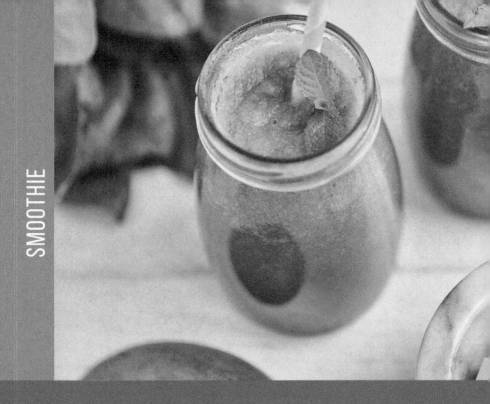

GREEN REVITALIZER SMOOTHIE

INGREDIENTS

- 4 large peeled kiwis
- 2 cups pineapple, diced
- 2 cups fresh baby spinach
- 2 cups almond milk
- 1 cup coconut water
- 2-inch piece of fresh peeled ginger
- Juice of 1 lime

DIRECTIONS

Add the ingredients in the order listed to a high-powered blender. Puree until thick and creamy. Serve your smoothie immediately and enjoy the refreshing fusion of kiwi, pineapple, spinach, and more.

NUTRITIONAL INFORMATION

Calories: 220 | Protein: 3g | Carbs: 45g | Fat: 5g

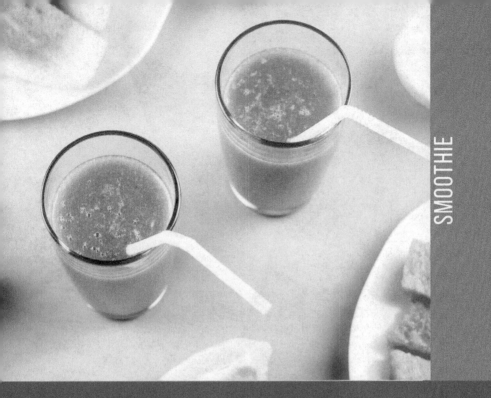

STRAWBERRY GRAPEFRUIT SMOOTHIE

INGREDIENTS

- 1 cup strawberry
- 2 ripe bananas
- 1 cup fresh orange or grapefruit
- 2 cups fresh grapefruit juice
- Honey, to taste

DIRECTIONS

Add all ingredients to your blender, creating a luscious and nutrient-rich base for your smoothie. Pour 2 cups of fresh grapefruit juice to infuse your smoothie with zesty and refreshing citrus flavors. Blend all the ingredients until they form a smooth and refreshing texture. Enjoy!

NUTRITIONAL INFORMATION

Calories: 220 | Protein: 2g | Carbs: 52g | Fat: 2g

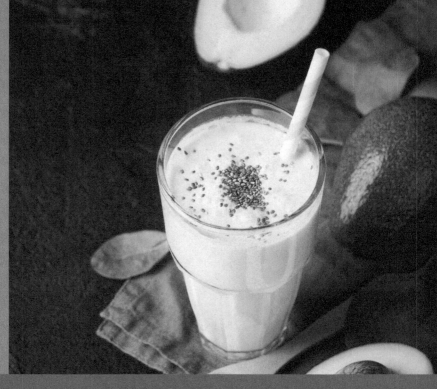

TROPICAL MORINGA SMOOTHIE

INGREDIENTS

- 1 ripe banana
- 1 avocado
- 2 cups mango chunks
- 1 cup baby spinach
- 1 and 1/2 cup coconut milk
- 1 tablespoon moringa powder
- 1 tablespoon almond butter (optional)

DIRECTIONS

Mix all ingredients in the blender until they form a smooth and rejuvenating texture. Taste your smoothie and adjust the sweetness or thickness by adding more banana or coconut milk, if needed. Serve your smoothie immediately, and enjoy!

NUTRITIONAL INFORMATION

Calories: 310 | Protein: 5g | Carbs: 31g | Fat: 21g

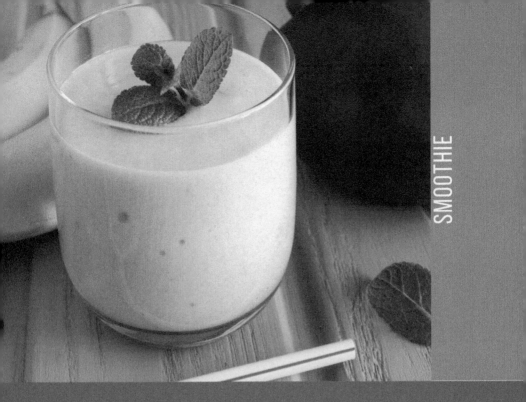

MANGO-MANGO SMOOTHIE

INGREDIENTS

- 1 ripe banana
- 3 cups mango chunks
- 2 cups coconut water
- 1 tablespoon mangosteen powder
- Honey, to taste

DIRECTIONS

Add the ingredients in the order listed to a high-powered blender. Puree until thick and creamy. Serve your smoothie immediately and enjoy the refreshing mango and coconut water fusion.

NUTRITIONAL INFORMATION

Calories: 260 | Protein: 3g | Carbs: 61g | Fat: 2g

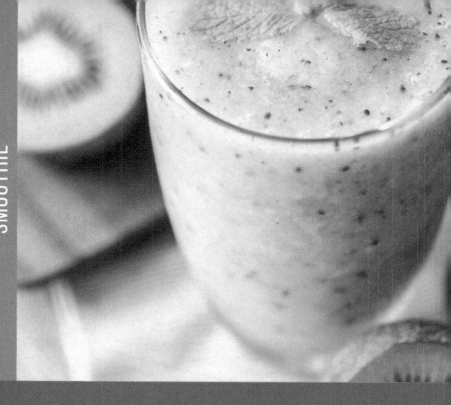

SMOOTHIE

MATCHA MINT SMOOTHIE

INGREDIENTS

- 4 big peeled kiwis
- 1 ripe banana
- 1 cup cashew milk
- 1 tablespoon honey
- 1 cup baby spinach
- 1/4 cup fresh mint leaves
- 1 tablespoon hulled hemp seeds
- 1 teaspoon matcha powder

DIRECTIONS

Add the ingredients in the order listed to a high-powered blender. Puree until thick and creamy. Taste your smoothie and adjust the sweetness or consistency by adding more honey or cashew milk if needed. Serve your smoothie immediately, and enjoy!

NUTRITIONAL INFORMATION

Calories: 425 | Protein: 7g | Carbs: 71g | Fat: 15g

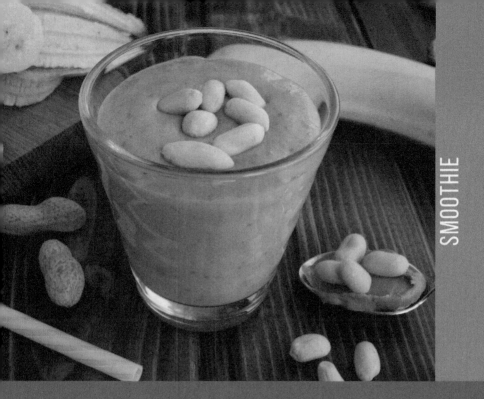

PEANUT BUTTER AND BERRY SMOOTHIE

INGREDIENTS

- 4 oz acai puree
- 1 ripe banana
- 1/2 cup peanut butter
- 1 cup mixed berries (strawberries, blueberries, and raspberries)
- 1 cup cashew milk

DIRECTIONS

Blend all the ingredients until your smoothie reaches a velvety texture and all components are thoroughly combined. Taste the smoothie and adjust the sweetness or consistency by adding more peanut butter or cashew milk, if desired. Enjoy!

NUTRITIONAL INFORMATION

Calories: 621 | Protein: 20g | Carbs: 49g | Fat: 42g

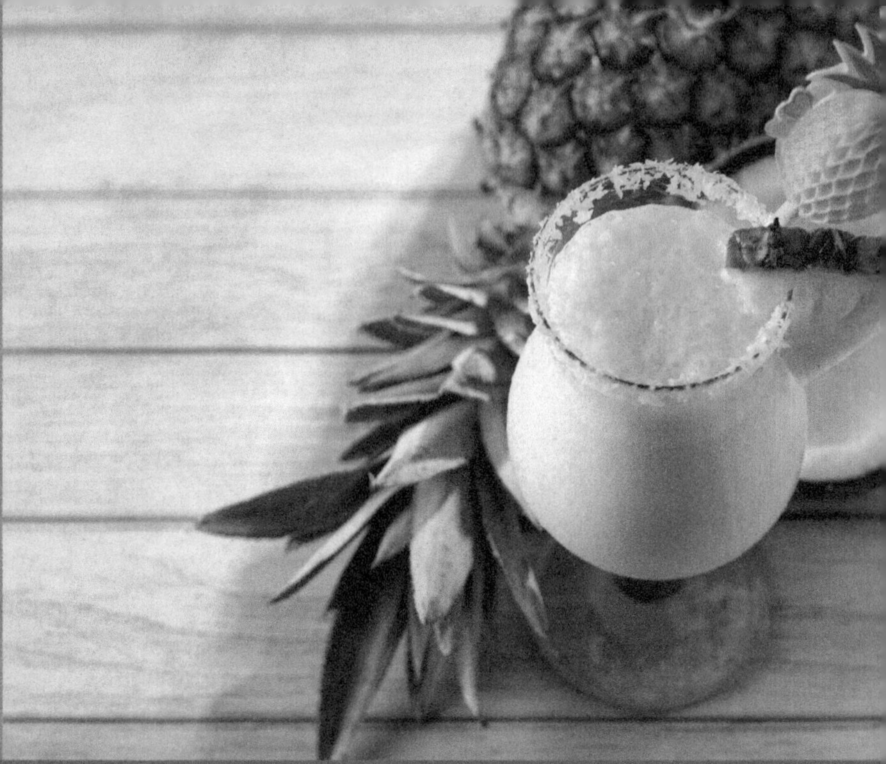

SMOOTHIE

SPICY PINEAPPLE SMOOTHIE

INGREDIENTS

- 3.5 oz apple puree
- 1 cup pineapple chunks
- 1 ripe banana
- 2 cups coconut water
- 1/4 teaspoon cayenne powder

DIRECTIONS

Blend all the ingredients until your Spicy Pineapple Smoothie reaches a smooth and well-combined texture. Taste the smoothie and adjust the spiciness by adding more or less cayenne powder if desired. Serve and enjoy!

NUTRITIONAL INFORMATION

Calories: 315 | Protein: 3g | Carbs: 77g | Fat: 2g

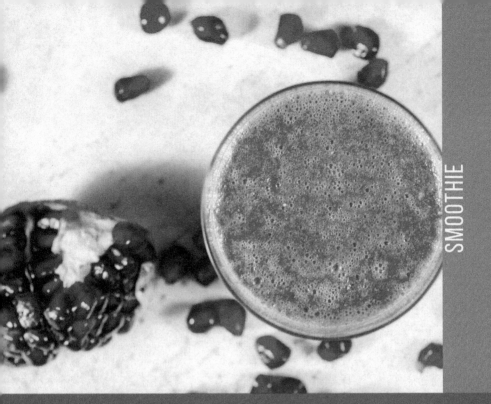

PROTEIN & POMEGRANATE SMOOTHIE

INGREDIENTS

- 4 oz mixed berries
- 1 scoop vanilla-flavored protein powder
- 1 cup vanilla-flavored almond milk
- 1/2 cup pomegranate juice
- 1/2 banana
- 1 tablespoon almond butter
- 1 tablespoon honey
- Pomegranate seeds for garnish

DIRECTIONS

Blend all the ingredients until your Spicy Pineapple Smoothie reaches a smooth and well-combined texture. Taste the smoothie and adjust the spiciness by adding more or less cayenne powder if desired. Serve and enjoy!

NUTRITIONAL INFORMATION

Calories: 315 | Protein: 3g | Carbs: 77g | Fat: 2g

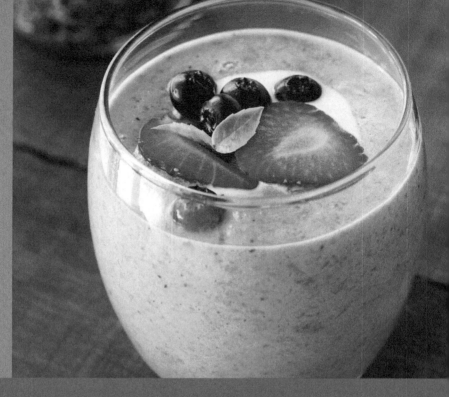

SMOOTHIE

BALSAMIC STRAWBERRY SMOOTHIE

INGREDIENTS

- 7 oz fresh strawberries
- 2 tablespoons pure maple syrup
- 1 tablespoon + 1 teaspoon balsamic vinegar
- 1 cup almond milk
- 1/3 cup Greek yogurt
- 1 banana
- 1/2 teaspoon cardamom powder

DIRECTIONS

Add the ingredients in the order listed to a high-powered blender. Puree until thick and creamy. Add more maple syrup or milk to taste your smoothie and adjust the sweetness or consistency. Serve your smoothie immediately, and enjoy!

NUTRITIONAL INFORMATION

Calories: 315 | Protein: 3g | Carbs: 77g | Fat: 2g

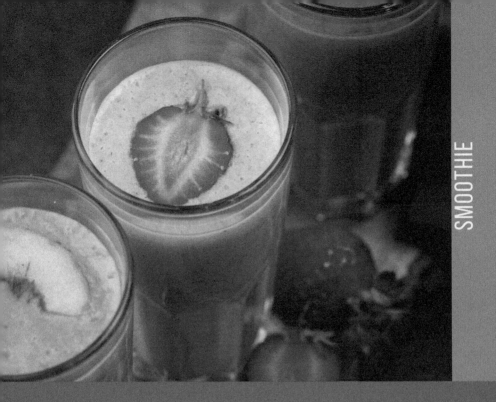

STRAWBERRY BANANA SMOOTHIE

INGREDIENTS

- 1 banana
- 3 cups strawberries
- 2 cups vanilla-flavored cashew milk
- 2 tablespoons baobab powder

DIRECTIONS

Add the ingredients in the order listed to a high-powered blender. Puree until thick and creamy. Your Strawberry Banana Smoothie is now ready to be enjoyed!

NUTRITIONAL INFORMATION

Calories: 320 | Protein: 6g | Carbs: 70g | Fat: 5g

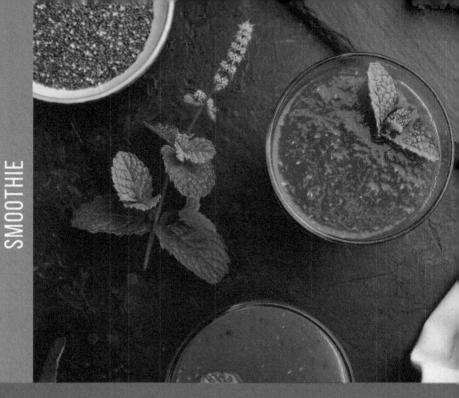

WATERMELON CHIA PUDDING

INGREDIENTS

- 7 oz acai puree
- 4 cups cubed watermelon
- 3 tablespoons chia seeds
- 2 tablespoons baobab powder
- 1 teaspoon lemon zest

DIRECTIONS

Blend all the necessary ingredients. Add chia seeds and baobab powder, providing a wonderful texture and plenty of fiber. Add lemon zest for a zesty touch, elevating the flavors and adding a refreshing hint. Transfer the mixture into serving glasses or jars. Cover and refrigerate for at least 2 hours or until the chia seeds have absorbed the liquid, creating a pudding-like consistency.

NUTRITIONAL INFORMATION

Calories: 315 | Protein: 3g | Carbs: 77g | Fat: 2g

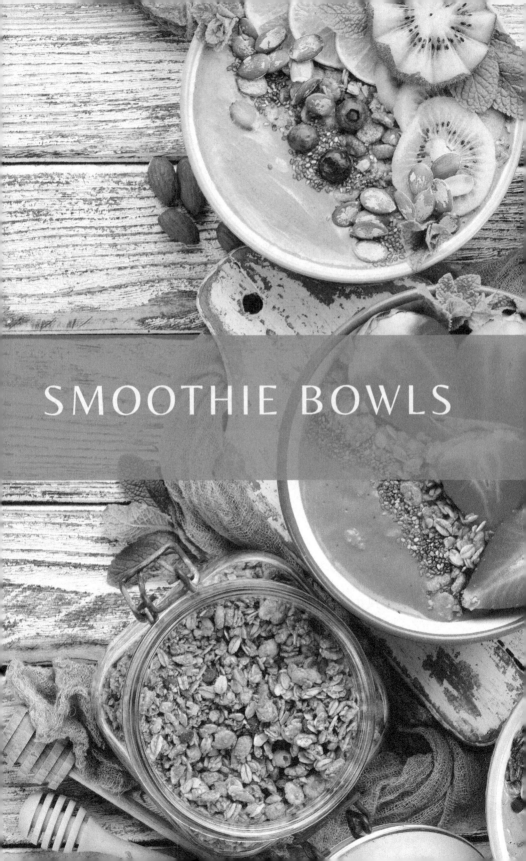

SMOOTHIE BOWLS

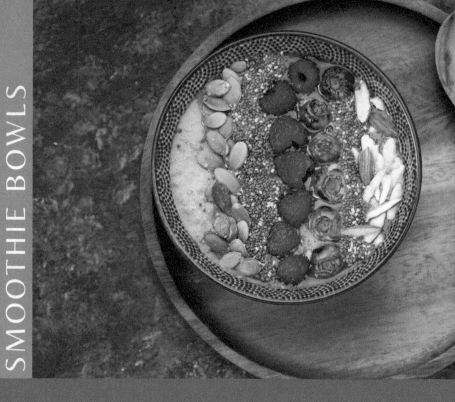

BERRY MANGO SMOOTHIE BOWL

INGREDIENTS

- 3.5 oz guava puree
- 1/2 cup mixed berries
- 3/4 cup almond milk
- 1 cup mango
- 1/2 banana
- 3/4 cup coconut water
- Optional toppings:
- 1/2 cup blueberries
- 1/2 cup raspberries
- 1/2 cup coconut flakes
- 1/2 cup granola
- Sprinkle of chia seeds

DIRECTIONS

Prepare your Berry Mango Smoothie Bowl by blending guava puree, mixed berries, almond milk, mango, banana, and coconut water. Once smooth, transfer to a bowl, then top with granola, blueberries, raspberries, coconut flakes, and chia seeds. Arrange these toppings to your liking for a vibrant and delicious start to your day.

NUTRITIONAL INFORMATION

Calories: 350 | Protein: 5g | Carbs: 70g | Fat: 8g

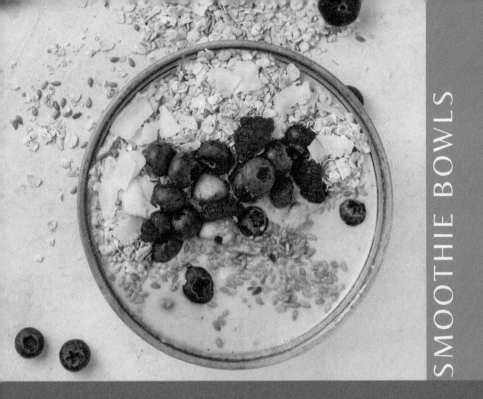

BRIGHT OATMEAL BOWL

INGREDIENTS

- 4 oz acai or guava puree
- 1 banana
- 1/4 cup oats
- 4 Medjool dates, pitted
- 2 tablespoons cacao nibs
- 2 tablespoons coconut flakes
- 2 tablespoons almond butter
- Optional toppings:
- 2 tablespoons oats
- 2 tablespoons cacao nibs
- Fresh blueberries
- Raspberries

DIRECTIONS

Blend acai or guava puree, banana, oats, Medjool dates, cacao nibs, coconut flakes, and almond butter to make your Bright Oatmeal Bowl. Once blended, transfer to a bowl and top with oats, cacao nibs, blueberries, and raspberries for added flavor and texture. Enjoy this nutritious and flavorful bowl to kickstart your day.

NUTRITIONAL INFORMATION

Calories: 350 | Protein: 5g | Carbs: 70g | Fat: 8g

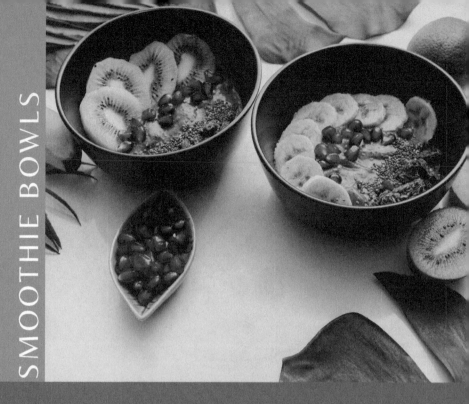

PUMPKIN SPICE SMOOTHIE BOWL

INGREDIENTS

- 1 banana
- 2 cups pumpkin puree
- 2 cups chopped apple
- 2 tablespoons almond butter
- 1 teaspoon cinnamon
- 1 teaspoon turmeric
- 1/4 teaspoon ground nutmeg
- 1/2 cup almond milk
- Topping:
- 2 tablespoons pumpkin seeds
- 2 tablespoons pomegranate

DIRECTIONS

For a Pumpkin Spice Smoothie Bowl, blend banana, pumpkin puree, chopped apple, almond butter, spices, and almond milk. Pour into a bowl and top with pumpkin seeds, pomegranate arils, and a sliced banana for a delightful fall treat. Enjoy the rich and comforting flavors with every spoonful.

NUTRITIONAL INFORMATION

Calories: 510 | Protein: 9g | Carbs: 81g | Fat: 18g |

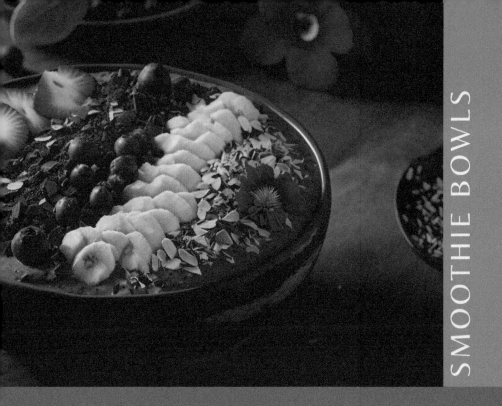

CHOCOLATE PROTEIN SMOOTHIE BOWL

INGREDIENTS

- 4 oz fruit puree
- 1 banana
- 1 cup blackberries
- 2 scoops chocolate-flavored protein powder
- 1 tablespoon cacao powder
- 1 tablespoon maca powder
- 1 cup almond milk
- Topping:
- 1 cup mixed berries
- 2 tablespoons cacao nibs
- Sprinkle of coconut flakes or granola

DIRECTIONS

Blend all ingredients. Once blended, transfer to a bowl and top with cacao nibs, blueberries, and raspberries for added flavor and texture. Sprinkle the bowl of coconut flakes or granola. Enjoy this nutritious and flavorful bowl to kickstart your day.

NUTRITIONAL INFORMATION

Calories: 470 | Protein: 29g | Carbs: 57g | Fat: 15g |

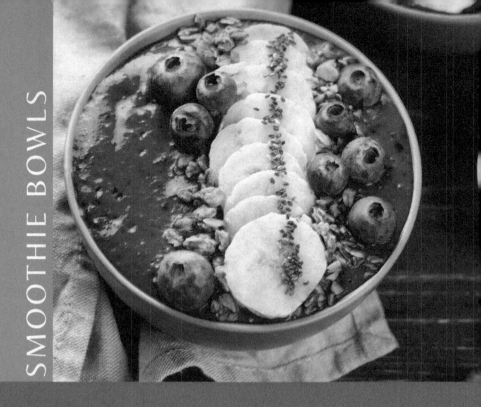

PROTEIN-PACKED SUPERFOOD BOWL

INGREDIENTS

- 1 banana
- 1 cup blueberries
- 1 cup mango
- 2 scoops protein powder
- 2 teaspoons spirulina powder
- 2 teaspoons mangosteen
- 1 and 1/2 cup almond milk
- Toppings:
- 1 cup fresh fruits and berries
- 1 banana
- 2 tablespoons sunflower seeds
- Chia seeds

DIRECTIONS

Prepare your toppings by slicing the banana and gathering fresh fruits, berries, sunflower seeds, and chia seeds. Blend banana, blueberries, mango, protein powder, spirulina, mangosteen powder, and almond milk until creamy. Pour into a bowl and decorate with the prepared toppings. Indulge in your Protein-Packed Superfood Smoothie Bowl for a nourishing breakfast or energizing snack.

NUTRITIONAL INFORMATION

Calories: 470 | Protein: 29g | Carbs: 57g | Fat: 15g |

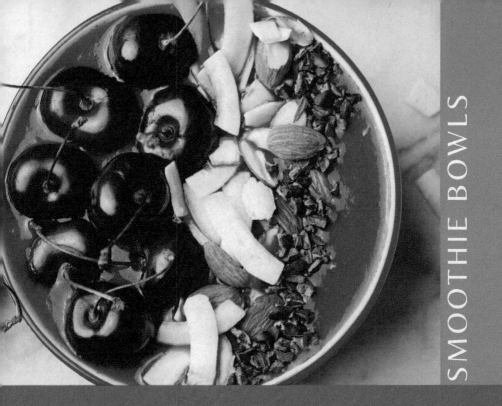

CHOCOLATE-CHERRY SMOOTHIE BOWL

INGREDIENTS

- 4 oz beloved fruit puree
- 1 banana
- 1 cup pitted sweet cherries
- 2 scoops chocolate-flavored protein powder
- 1/4 cup dark cacao powder
- 1 cup vanilla-flavored almond or cashew milk
- Toppings:
- 2 cups cherries
- 1/4 cup cacao nibs
- 1/4 cup raw almonds
- 1/4 cup coconut flakes

DIRECTIONS

Prepare your toppings by washing cherries, toasting coconut flakes, and gathering cacao nibs and raw almonds. Blend fruit puree, banana, pitted sweet cherries, protein powder, dark cacao powder, and almond or cashew milk. Pour into a bowl and top with fresh cherries, cacao nibs, almonds, and toasted coconut flakes. Enjoy the decadent Chocolate-Cherry Smoothie Bowl, a delightful and nutritious treat.

NUTRITIONAL INFORMATION

Calories: 685 | Protein: 32g | Carbs: 90g | Fat: 29g |

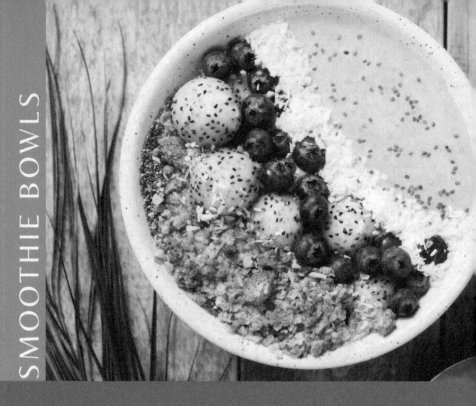

SMOOTHIE BOWLS

BLUE SPIRULINA SMOOTHIE BOWL

INGREDIENTS

- 4 oz berry puree
- 2 bananas
- 1/2 cup green grapes
- 2 teaspoons spirulina powder
- 1 can cream of coconut
- Toppings:
- 1/2 cup blackberries
- 1/2 cup blueberries
- 1/2 dragon fruit

DIRECTIONS

Prepare your toppings by rinsing the blackberries and blueberries and slicing the dragon fruit. Combine berry puree, bananas, green grapes, spirulina powder, and cream of coconut. Blend until smooth and vibrant. Pour into a bowl, topping the Spirulina Superfood Smoothie Bowl with blackberries, blueberries, and dragon fruit. Enjoy this nutrient-rich and visually stunning creation.

NUTRITIONAL INFORMATION

Calories: 646 | Protein: 6g | Carbs: 102g | Fat: 26g |

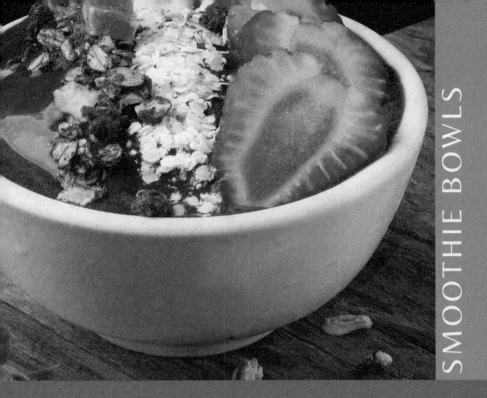

CHOCOLATE STRAWBERRY PROTEIN BOWL

INGREDIENTS

- 7 oz acai puree
- 2 cups strawberries
- 2 scoops chocolate-flavored protein powder
- 1 tablespoon dark cacao powder
- Chocolate-flavored almond milk
- Toppings:
- 1 cup sliced strawberries
- 1/2 cup chocolate granola
- 2 tablespoons coconut flakes

DIRECTIONS

Blend acai puree, strawberries, chocolate-flavored protein powder, and dark cacao powder in a high-speed blender. Adjust the consistency with chocolate-flavored almond milk and blend until smooth. Serve the chocolate-covered strawberry smoothie in a bowl, topping it with sliced strawberries, chocolate granola, and coconut flakes. This protein-rich bowl is ideal for a delicious treat and post-workout recovery.

NUTRITIONAL INFORMATION

Calories: 548 | Protein: 38g | Carbs: 77g | Fat: 15g |

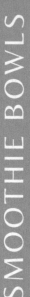

SMOOTHIE BOWLS

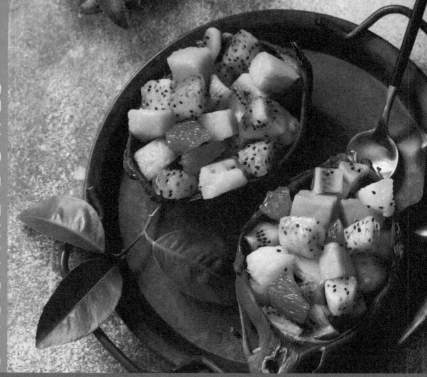

TROPICAL PARADISE ACAI BOWL

INGREDIENTS

- 7 oz acai puree
- 1 banana
- 1 cup papaya chunks
- 2 kiwi
- 1/4 cup fresh mint leaves
- 1/4 cup fresh lime juice
- 1 cup almond milk
- Toppings:
- 1 dragon fruit, cut in half lengthwise, seeds removed, and flesh scooped out
- 1/2 cup chanks orange
- 2 tablespoons nuts
- 1 kiwi, peeled and sliced

DIRECTIONS

Combine acai puree, banana, papaya, kiwi, mint, lime juice, and almond milk until smooth. Pour the tropical mixture into a bowl and top it with papaya, berries, kiwi, and chopped nuts for a refreshing Tropical Paradise Acai Bowl, a feast for your taste buds. Enjoy your taste of the tropics!

NUTRITIONAL INFORMATION

Calories: 487 | Protein: 8g | Carbs: 97g | Fat: 10g |

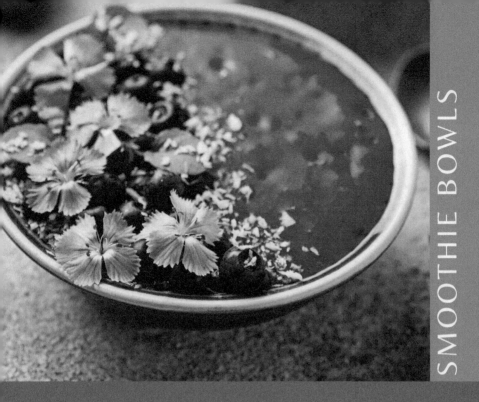

MIXED BERRY BOWL

INGREDIENTS

- 7 oz acai puree
- 1 banana
- 1 cup mixed berries (strawberries, blueberries, raspberries, blackberries)
- 1 cup coconut water
- Topping:
- 1/2 cup fresh blueberries
- 1/2 cup raspberries or blackberries
- 1/2 cup coconut flakes
- 1/2 cup granola

DIRECTIONS

Combine acai puree, banana, mixed berries, and coconut water in a blender until smooth. Pour the mixture into a bowl and top it with fresh berries, coconut flakes, and granola for a flavorful Mixed Berry Acai Bowl. Delight in this healthy and delicious creation!

NUTRITIONAL INFORMATION

Calories: 495 | Protein: 5g | Carbs: 87g | Fat: 17g |

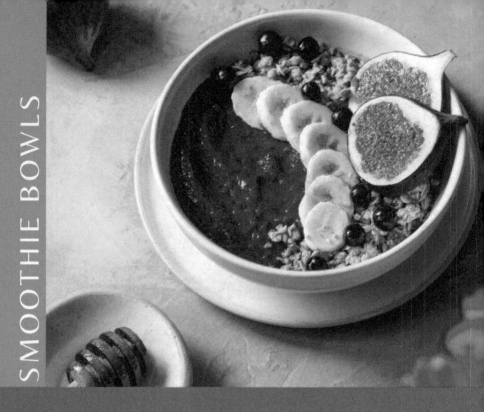

FIG AND BLUEBERRY BOWL

INGREDIENTS

- 5 peeled kiwis
- 1 and 1/2 cups blueberries
- 1 and 1/2 cups baby spinach
- 4 fresh figs
- 1/2 cup non-fat Greek yogurt
- 1/4 cup almond milk
- Topping:
- 4 fresh figs
- 1/2 cup berries
- 1/2 cup granola

DIRECTIONS

Combine kiwis, blueberries, baby spinach, figs, Greek yogurt, and almond milk in a blender until smooth. Pour the mixture into a bowl and top it with fresh figs, raspberries, and granola for a tasty Fig and Blueberry Bowl. Enjoy this nutritious and delicious creation!

NUTRITIONAL INFORMATION

Calories: 480 | Protein: 11g | Carbs: 98g | Fat: 7g |

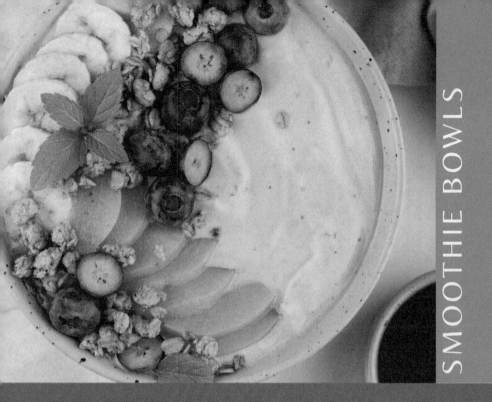

PEACH DELIGHT BOWL

INGREDIENTS

- 3.5 oz acai puree
- 2 cups peach slices
- 1 tablespoon maple syrup
- 1 teaspoon vanilla extract
- 1/2 teaspoon ground cinnamon
- 3/4 cup coconut yogurt
- Topping:
- 1 and 1/2 cups sliced peaches
- 1 cup almond granola
- 1 banana
- 1/2 cup berries

DIRECTIONS

Combine all ingredients in a high-speed blender. Blend until you achieve a smooth and creamy consistency. Top your bowl with sliced peaches and a generous sprinkle of almond granola, berries and banana. Serve and enjoy your nutritious and delicious creation!

NUTRITIONAL INFORMATION

Calories: 540 | Protein: 5g | Carbs: 86g | Fat: 22g |

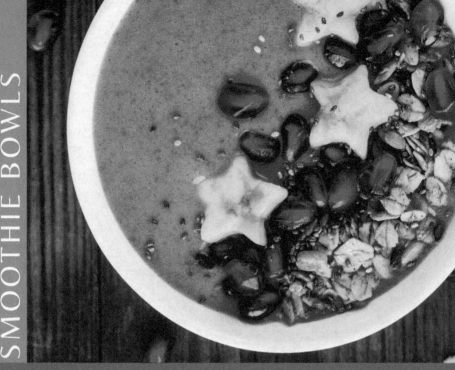

TROPICAL MANGO BLISS BOWL

INGREDIENTS

- 3.5 oz guava puree
- 1 cup mango chunks
- 1 cup pineapple chunks
- 1 teaspoon mangosteen powder
- 1 cup coconut milk
- Topping:
- 1/2 cup sliced mango
- 1/2 cup berries
- 1/4 cup pomegranate arils
- 1/4 cup granola

DIRECTIONS

Combine guava puree, mango, pineapple, mangosteen powder, and coconut milk in a blender until smooth. Pour the mixture into a bowl and top it with sliced mango, berries, pomegranate arils, coconut, granola and fresh mint leaves. Enjoy the Tropical Mango Bliss Acai Bowl for a delightful tropical escape!

NUTRITIONAL INFORMATION

Calories: 525 | Protein: 5g | Carbs: 68g | Fat: 29g |

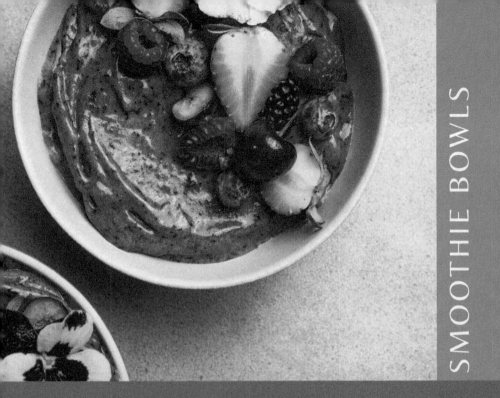

BLACKBERRY ACAI BOWL

INGREDIENTS

- 3.5 oz acai puree
- 1 banana
- 1 and 1/2 cup blackberries
- 2 tablespoons flaxseed meal
- 2 teaspoons rosewater
- 1/2 cup almond milk
- Topping:
- 1/2 cup blackberries
- 1/4 cup mixed berries
- 1/4 cup mulberries

DIRECTIONS

Combine acai puree, banana, blackberries, flaxseed meal, rosewater, and almond milk in a blender for a smooth mixture. Pour the blend into a bowl and top with remaining blackberries, mixed berries, mulberries, and a sprinkle of flaxseed. The addition of rosewater offers a subtle floral note to this delightful and unique Blackberry Acai Bowl. Enjoy the sweet, earthy, and floral flavors in every spoonful. Serve this bowl for a lovely breakfast or snack.

NUTRITIONAL INFORMATION

Calories: 358 | Protein: 8g | Carbs: 64g | Fat: 11g |

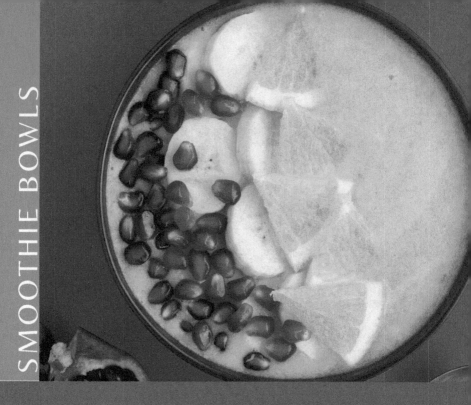

CANTALOUPE SUNRISE BOWL

INGREDIENTS

- 7 oz fruit puree
- 2 cups chopped cantaloupe
- 1 teaspoon flaxseed meal
- 1/2 cup cashew milk
- Topping:
- 1/4 goji berries or pomegranate
- 1 tablespoon hemp hearts
- slices orange
- Fresh strawberries
- banana
- Coconut flakes

DIRECTIONS

Combine fruit puree, cantaloupe, flaxseed meal, and cashew milk in a blender for a creamy base. Pour the blend into a bowl and top it with goji berries, hemp hearts, fresh cantaloupe balls, strawberries, and coconut flakes. The mix of sweet cantaloupe and fruit puree creates a delightful flavor contrast. Enjoy the refreshing and fruity goodness of this Cantaloupe Sunrise Acai Bowl for a lovely breakfast.

NUTRITIONAL INFORMATION

Calories: 358 | Protein: 8g | Carbs: 64g | Fat: 11g |

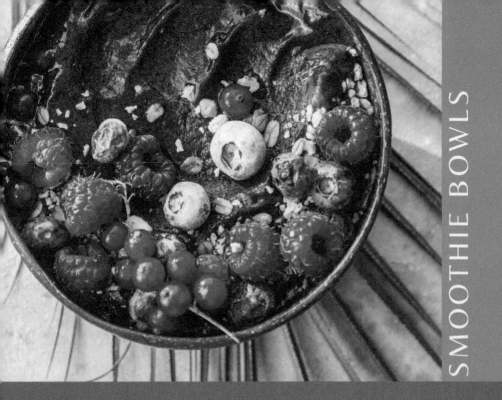

RASPBERRY CHOCO-CHIA BOWL

INGREDIENTS

- 4 oz berry puree
- 1 and 1/2 cups raspberries
- 1 tablespoon cacao powder
- 1 tablespoon chia seeds
- 3/4 cup almond milk
- Topping:
- 1/2 cup raspberries
- 1/2 mixed berries
- 1 tablespoon chia seeds
- 1 tablespoon cacao nibs
- 1/4 cup nuts

DIRECTIONS

Blend berry puree, raspberries, cacao powder, chia seeds, and almond milk for a smooth, creamy base. Pour it into a bowl and top it with raspberries, chia seeds, berries and cacao nibs for texture and flavor. The mix of sweet raspberries and chocolatey cacao creates a delicious bowl. Serve and relish the delightful taste of your Raspberry Choco-Chia Bowl.

NUTRITIONAL INFORMATION

Calories: 347 | Protein: 7g | Carbs: 48g | Fat: 17g |

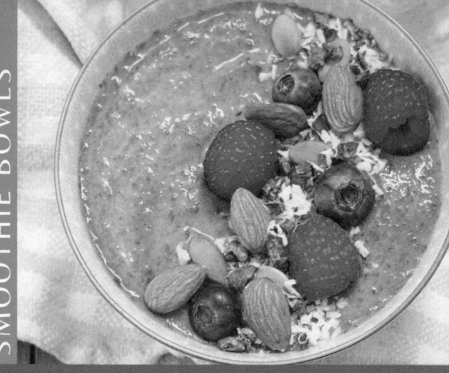

GREEN ENERGY BOWL

INGREDIENTS

- 7 oz kiwi puree
- 2 cups baby kale
- 1 cup baby spinach
- 2 bananas
- 1/2 teaspoon spirulina powder
- 1 cup coconut milk
- Topping:
- 1 banana, sliced
- 1/4 cup raw almonds
- 1/2 cup mixed berries
- 1/4 cup pumpkin or sunflower seeds
- 1/4 cup flaked coconut

DIRECTIONS

Combine kiwi puree, baby kale, baby spinach, bananas, spirulina powder, and coconut milk in a blender for a smooth green base. Once poured into a bowl, top it with banana slices, raw almonds, mixed berries, pumpkin seeds, and flaked coconut for various textures and flavors. This nutritious and refreshing bowl is an ideal start to your day. Serve and enjoy your Green Energy Bowl!

NUTRITIONAL INFORMATION

Calories: 647 | Protein: 15g | Carbs: 81g | Fat: 34g |

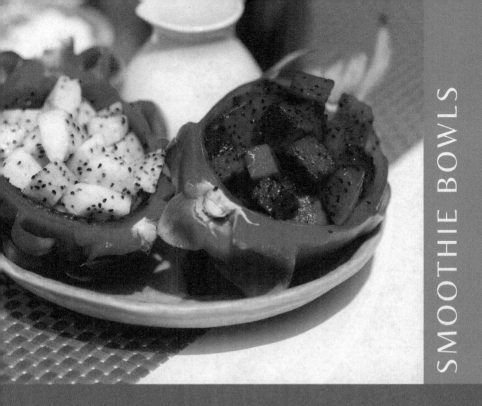

DRAGON FRUIT BOWL

INGREDIENTS

- 7 oz mixed beries
- 1 packed dragon fruit
- 2 bananas
- 1/4 cup vanilla-flavored protein powder
- 1 scoop baobab powder
- 1/2 cup cashew milk
- Topping:
- 1/2 cup coconut yogurt
- 1/2 cup chopped red and white dragon fruit
- 1/2 cup granola

DIRECTIONS

To prepare the bowl base, blend all ingredients. Once poured into a bowl, top it with creamy coconut yogurt and chopped red and white dragon fruit for a tropical twist. Finish with a layer of granola for added texture. Your Dragon Fruit Acai Bowl is ready to serve. Enjoy this visually stunning and nutritious creation!

NUTRITIONAL INFORMATION

Calories: 795 | Protein: 29g | Carbs: 127g | Fat: 24g |

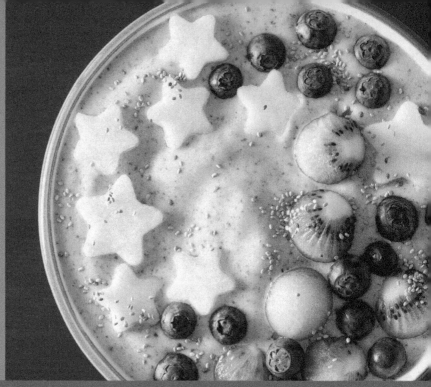

GREEN PLEASURE BOWL

INGREDIENTS

- 4 large peeled kiwis
- 2 bananas
- 1 cup green grapes
- 1 cup baby spinach
- 1 teaspoon spirulina powder
- 1/2 avocado
- 1 cup almond milk
- Topping:
- 1/4 cup sliced kiwi
- Sprinkle of whole oats
- 1 cup green grapes, sliced

1 tablespoon chia seeds

DIRECTIONS

To create your Green Pleasure Bowl, blend kiwis, bananas, green grapes, spinach, spirulina, avocado, and almond milk until smooth. Pour this vibrant mixture into a bowl. Top it with sliced green grapes, chia seeds, sliced kiwi, and a sprinkle of whole oats for a refreshing and nutritious morning treat. Enjoy the contrasting flavors and textures in this delightful bowl!

NUTRITIONAL INFORMATION

Calories: 590 | Protein: 8g | Carbs: 108g | Fat: 18g

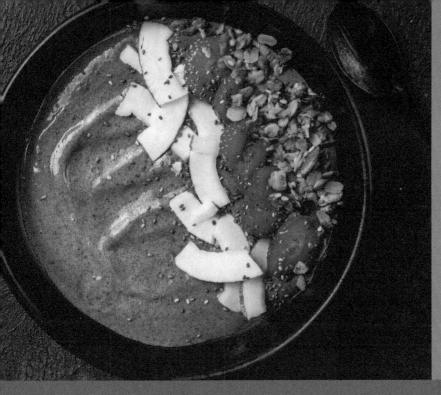

PEANUT BUTTER PARADISE BOWL

INGREDIENTS

- 7 oz guava puree
- 1 banana
- 3 tablespoons peanut butter
- 1/2 cup coconut milk
- 1 cup baby spinach
- 1/4 cup mixed berries
- Topping:
- 1 banana
- 2 tablespoons shredded coconut
- 2 tablespoons hulled hemp seeds

DIRECTIONS

To prepare your Peanut Butter Paradise Bowl, blend guava puree, banana, peanut butter, coconut milk, spinach, and mixed berries until smooth. Pour the creamy mixture into a bowl, then top it with sliced banana, shredded coconut, and hulled hemp seeds. Indulge in the creamy, nutty delight with every spoonful!

NUTRITIONAL INFORMATION

Calories: 590 | Protein: 8g | Carbs: 108g | Fat: 18g

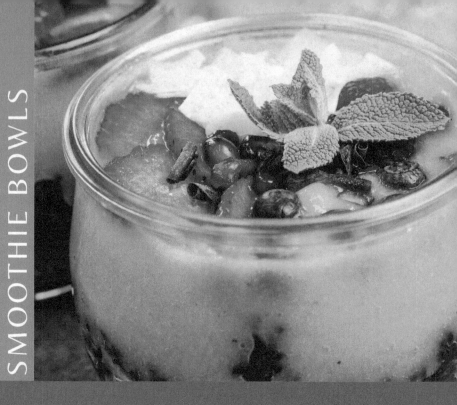

SMOOTHIE BOWLS

MANGO TURMERIC BOWL

INGREDIENTS

- 4 oz fruit puree
- 1 cup mango chunks
- 1 seedless navel orange, peeled
- 2 teaspoons turmeric powder
- 1 teaspoon chia seeds
- 1 and 1/2 cups kefir
- Topping:
- 1/2 sliced peach or nectarine
- 1/2 cup mixed berries
- 1 teaspoon chia seeds
- 2 tablespoons kefir

DIRECTIONS

Combine fruit puree, mango chunks, an orange, turmeric powder, chia seeds, and kefir in a blender until smooth. Pour this vibrant blend into a bowl and top it with sliced peach, mixed berries, and a drizzle of kefir. Add a final touch of chia seeds for a nutritious Mango Turmeric Bowl ready to be savored!

NUTRITIONAL INFORMATION

Calories: 430 | Protein: 9g | Carbs: 70g | Fat: 13g |

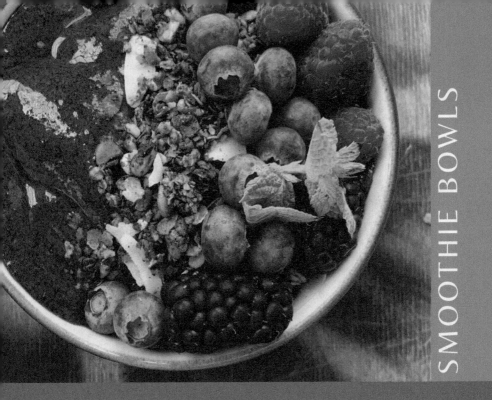

BLUEBERRY MACA PROTEIN BOWL

INGREDIENTS

- 2 cups blueberries
- 1 banana
- 1 cup mixed berries
- 2 scoops vanilla-flavored protein powder
- 2 tablespoons maca powder
- 3/4 cup macadamia nut milk
- Topping:
- 1 cup blueberries
- 1/4 cup chopped macadamia nuts
- Sprinkle of chia seeds

DIRECTIONS

Combine berries, bananas, vanilla protein powder, maca, and macadamia milk in a blender. Pour the mixture into a bowl and top it with extra blueberries, chopped macadamia nuts, and a sprinkle of chia seeds for a delicious and nutritious Blueberry Maca Protein Acai Bowl to start your day!

NUTRITIONAL INFORMATION

Calories: 500 | Protein: 30g | Carbs: 70g | Fat: 14g |

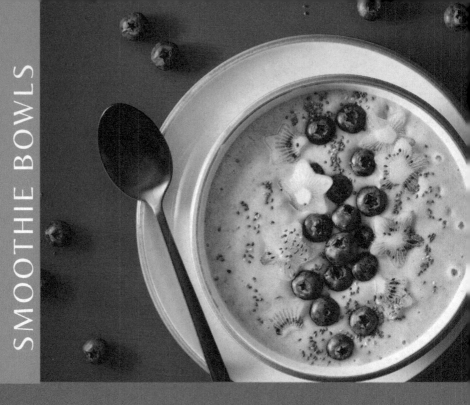

COLOR BERRIES & DRAGON FRUIT BOWL

INGREDIENTS

- 7 oz acai puree
- 2 bananas
- 2 tablespoons hemp seeds
- 2 tablespoons chia seeds
- 1/2 cup coconut milk
- 1 teaspoon spirulina
- 1 teaspoon butterfly pea powder
- Topping:
- 1/2 cup chopped dragon
- 1/2 cup blackberries
- 1/4 cup peeled chopped kiwi
- 1/4 cup crushed goji berries

DIRECTIONS

Blend acai puree, bananas, hulled hemp seeds, chia seeds, coconut milk, spirulina powder, and butterfly pea powder until smooth. Pour the mix into a bowl and top it with chopped dragon fruit, blackberries, kiwi, and crushed goji berries for a vibrant Dragon fruit Bliss Acai Bowl. Experience a delightful blend of taste and color!

NUTRITIONAL INFORMATION

Calories: 540 | Protein: 12g | Carbs: 80g | Fat: 22g |

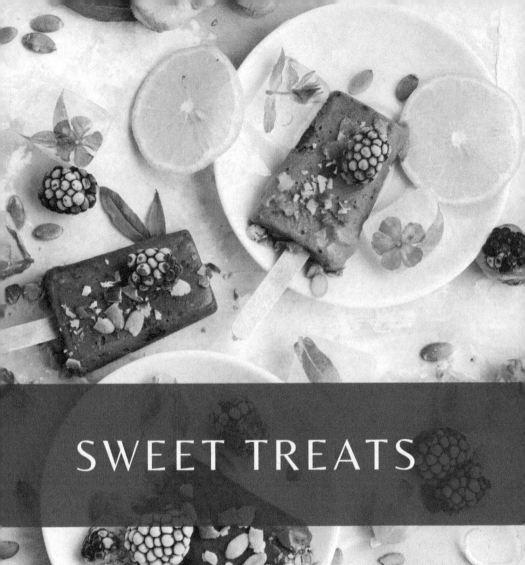

SWEET TREATS

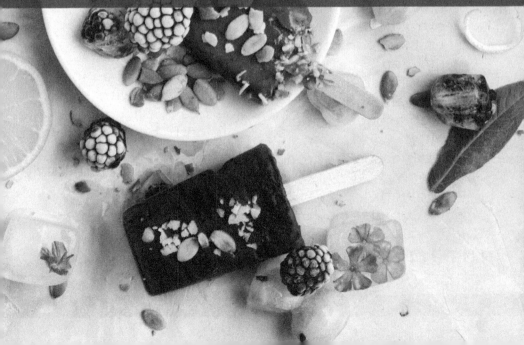

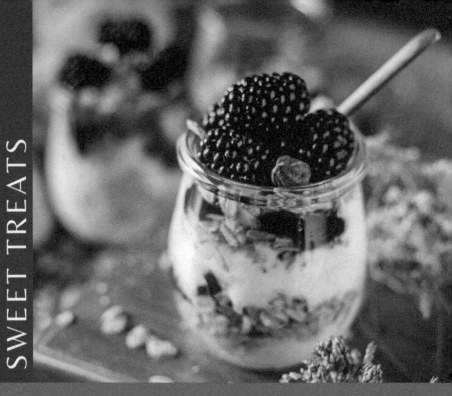

SWEET TREATS

PARFAIT WITH MIXED BERRIES

INGREDIENTS

- 1/4 cup chia seeds
- 1 and 1/4 cups cashew milk
- 1 teaspoon vanilla extract
- 1 tablespoon acai powder
- 1 cup fresh mixed berries
- 1 banana
- 1 tablespoon almond butter
- 2 tablespoons shredded coconut
- Topping:
- 1/2 cup granola
- 1/2 cup mixed berries

DIRECTIONS

Combine chia seeds, cashew milk, vanilla extract, and acai powder, ensuring an even distribution. Refrigerate for at least 4 hours. When ready, layer the acai chia pudding with mixed berries, sliced banana, almond butter, shredded coconut, and granola for a delightful Acai Parfait with Mixed Berries, blending textures and flavors.

NUTRITIONAL INFORMATION

Calories: 570 | Protein: 10g | Carbohydrates: 68g | Fat: 31g

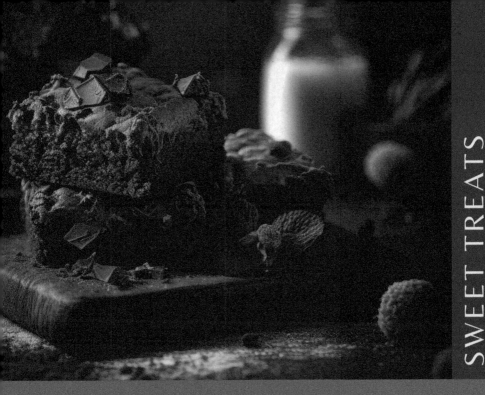

PROTEIN AND CACAO DARK BROWNIES

INGREDIENTS

- 2 cups ground oat flour
- 1/2 cup acai powder
- 1/2 cup raw cacao powder
- 1/4 cup vanilla-flavored protein powder
- 2/3 teaspoon baking soda
- Pinch of salt
- 2 cups canned pumpkin puree
- 2/3 cup maple syrup
- 2 tablespoons lemon juice
- 1/2 cup cacao nibs

DIRECTIONS

Preheat your oven to 350°F (175°C) and grease an 8x8-inch (20x20 cm) baking pan. Mix oat flour, acai powder, cacao, protein powder, baking soda, and salt in a bowl. Combine puree, syrup, and lemon juice in another bowl. Combine wet and dry ingredients, then fold in cacao nibs for added flavor and texture. Pour the batter into the prepared pan and bake for 25 min until a toothpick comes out clean. Cool the brownies, then cut them into 16 squares before serving. Enjoy!

NUTRITIONAL INFORMATION

Calories: 570 | Protein: 10g | Carbs: 68g | Fat: 31g |

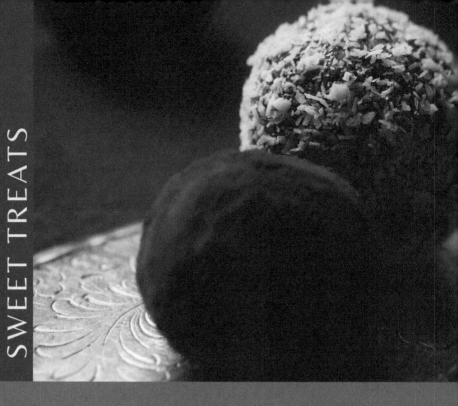

CACAO ENERGY BITES

INGREDIENTS

- 1 cup pitted and packed Medjool dates
- 2 cups raw walnuts
- 6 tablespoons cacao
- 1/2 teaspoon pink salt
- 3 tablespoons creamy almond butter
- 1 tablespoon melted coconut oil
- For Rolling:
- 2 tablespoons shredded coconut
- 2 tablespoons chopped walnuts
- 2 tablespoons cacao

DIRECTIONS

In a food processor, blend pitted Medjool dates until a sticky paste forms. Add raw walnuts and process until a coarse, crumb-like texture is achieved. Combine with cacao powder, pink Himalayan salt, almond butter, and melted coconut oil. Process until it turns sticky. Spread a mixture on a plate or tray. Shape small portions of the mixture into bite-sized balls and coat each in the cacao powder, coconut mixture, or chopped nuts. Place the coated bites on parchment paper and chill in the refrigerator for at least 30 minutes. Once firm, these Cacao Energy Bites are ready to provide a nutritious energy boost as a snack.

NUTRITIONAL INFORMATION

Calories: 116 |Fat: 7g | | Carbs: 13g | | Protein: 2g

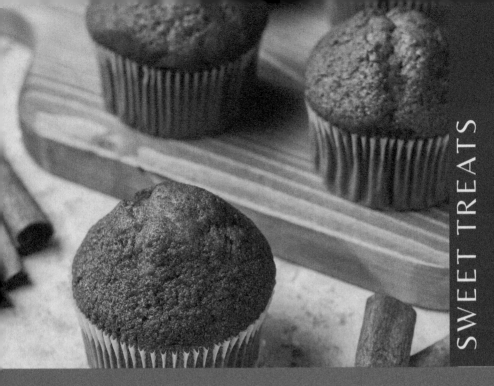

NUTRITION MORNING MUFFINS

INGREDIENTS

- 1 cup all-purpose flour
- 1/4 cup almond powder
- 1/2 teaspoon baking soda
- 1/2 teaspoon baking powder
- 3/4 teaspoon ground cinnamon
- 1/4 teaspoon ground ginger
- 1/8 teaspoon ground nutmeg
- 1/4 teaspoon kosher salt
- 1/4 cup coconut sugar
- 1 teaspoon vanilla extract
- 1 tablespoon melted coconut oil
- 2 eggs
- 3 tablespoons almond milk
- 1 cup shredded carrots
- 1/2 cup shredded zucchini
- 1/4 cup applesauce
- 1/4 cup golden raisins
- 3 tablespoons shredded coconut
- 2 tablespoons walnuts

DIRECTIONS

Preheat the oven to 350°F (175°C) and line a muffin tin with paper liners. Mix all-purpose flour, almond powder, baking soda, baking powder, ground cinnamon, ginger, nutmeg, and kosher salt in a medium-sized bowl. In another bowl, mix coconut sugar, vanilla extract, melted coconut oil, eggs, and almond milk until thoroughly combined. Combine the wet and dry mixtures. Gently fold in shredded carrots, zucchini, applesauce, golden raisins, coconut, and walnuts. Bake it 20 min. Cool the muffins in the tin, then transfer to a wire rack to cool completely.

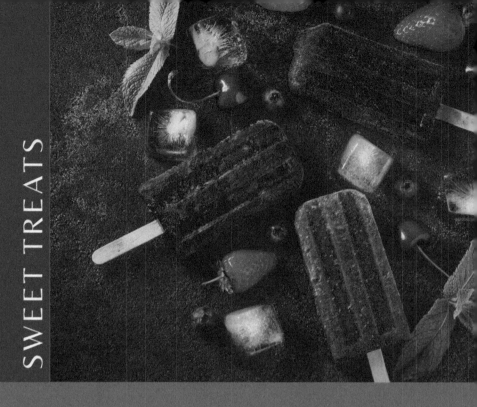

CHERRY CHIA ICE POPS

INGREDIENTS

- 1 cup vanilla-flavored almond milk
- 2 cups cherries
- 1 banana
- 3 tablespoons chia seeds

DIRECTIONS

Prepare your ice pop molds. Blend vanilla-flavored almond milk, cherries, and bananas until smooth. Transfer the mixture to a bowl or pitcher, then stir in the chia seeds. Pour the mix into the molds, leaving a small gap, and insert ice pop sticks. Freeze for at least 4 hours until solid. To serve, you can run the molds under warm water or remove disposable cups. Enjoy these nutritious Cherry Acai Chia Ice Pops!

NUTRITIONAL INFORMATION

Calories: 82 | Fat: 2g | Carbs: 16g | Protein: 2g

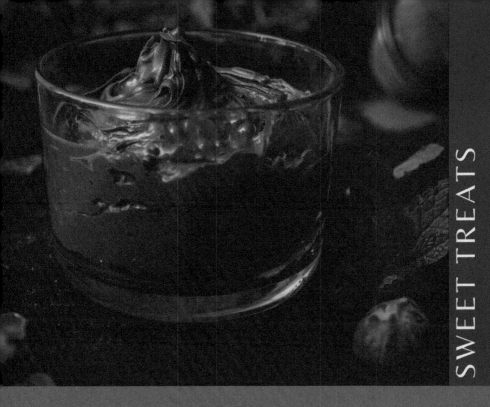

CHOCOLATE AVOCADO MOUSSE

INGREDIENTS

- 4 oz mango puree
- 1 avocado
- 1/4 cup cacao powder
- 2 bananas
- 2 tablespoons chocolate peanut butter
- 1/3 cup cashew milk

DIRECTIONS

Combine mango puree, ripe avocado, cacao powder, bananas, chocolate peanut butter, and cashew milk in a blender. Blend until smooth and creamy, scraping down the sides as needed. Adjust sweetness by adding more chocolate peanut butter if desired. Transfer the mousse to serving glasses, cover, and refrigerate for at least 2 hours. Garnish with chocolate shavings, fresh berries, or whipped coconut cream. Enjoy this satisfying and healthy dessert!

NUTRITIONAL INFORMATION

Calories: 82 | Fat: 2g | Carbs: 16g | Protein: 2g

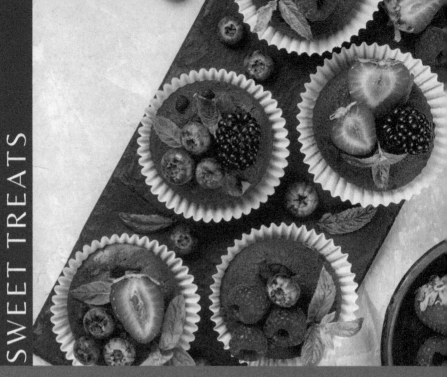

CUPCAKES & BUTTERCREAM FROSTING

INGREDIENTS

- For the Cupcakes:
- 1 and 1/2 cups caster sugar
- 1/2 cup unsalted butter, softened
- 3 eggs
- 1/2 cup boiling water
- 1 and 2/3 cups self-rising flour
- 1/2 cup dark cacao powder
- 1/2 teaspoon kosher salt
- 1 cup fresh blueberries
- For the Acai Buttercream Frosting:
- 2/3 cup unsalted butter, softened
- 2 and 1/2 cups confectioner's sugar
- 3 tablespoons acai powder
- 1/4 cup fresh berries (for decoration)

DIRECTIONS

Preheat the oven to 350°F (175°C) and line a muffin tin with 12 paper cupcake liners. Cream softened butter and caster sugar until fluffy; beat in eggs, then gradually add self-rising flour, dark cacao powder, kosher salt, and boiling water. Fold in fresh blueberries and bake for 20 minutes. Cool and transfer to a wire rack.

For the Buttercream Frosting: Beat softened butter, gradually add confectioner's sugar and acai powder until fluffy. Once cupcakes are cool, frost and decorate with fresh blueberries. Enjoy !

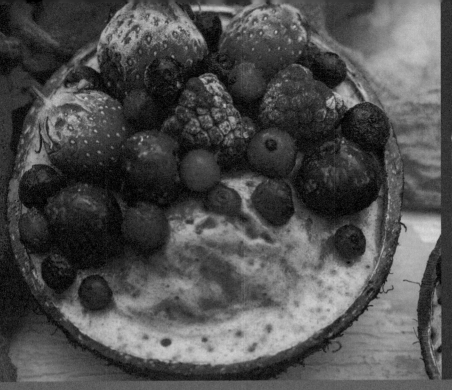

BLUEBERRY FROZEN YOGURT

INGREDIENTS

- 1 and 1/2 cups Greek yogurt
- 3/4 cup coconut sugar
- 4 cups fresh mixed berries
- 2 teaspoons lemon zest
- 2 teaspoons lemon juice

DIRECTIONS

Blend fresh berries, lemon zest, and juice until smooth. Whisk together Greek yogurt and coconut sugar until creamy. Gently fold the blueberry mixture into the sweetened Greek yogurt. Pour into a freezer-safe container and freeze for 4-6 hours or overnight. Before serving, briefly let it sit at room temperature. Scoop into bowls or cones top with fresh mixed berries, honey, or shredded coconut. Enjoy!

NUTRITIONAL INFORMATION

Calories: 263 |Fat: 7g | Carbs: 46g | Protein: 6g

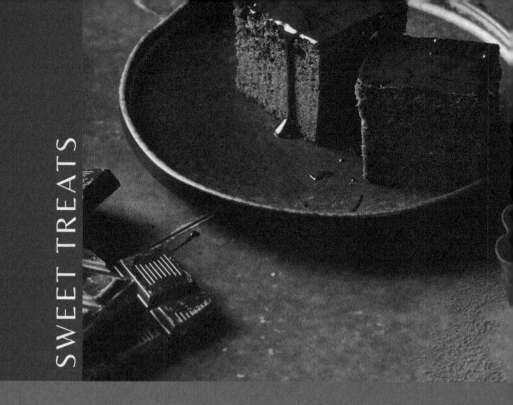

DARK CACAO FUDGE

INGREDIENTS

- 1/2 cup acai powder
- 3 tablespoons coconut oil
- 10 soft pitted Medjool dates
- 1/2 cup coconut or almond flour
- 1 teaspoon pink Himalayan salt
- 1 cup cacao butter
- 1 cup cacao paste
- 1/4 cup honey
- 1 teaspoon vanilla extract
- 1/2 cup pumpkin seeds

DIRECTIONS

Line a baking dish with parchment paper. Blend acai powder, coconut oil, dates, almond or coconut flour, and sea salt until smooth. Melt cacao butter and paste in a saucepan. Remove from heat, add honey, vanilla, and 1/4 teaspoon sea salt, whisking until combined. Optionally add pumpkin seeds. Pour half the chocolate mixture into the prepared pan. Shape the mixture by hand to fit the pan and place it on the chocolate layer. Pour the remaining chocolate over the acai layer and sprinkle 1/2 teaspoon salt. Freeze for 45 minutes to 1 hour, then cut into squares and serve.

NUTRITIONAL INFORMATION

Calories: 263 | Carbs: 46g | Protein: 6g | Fat: 7g

CONCLUSION

As you reach the end of "Healthy Smoothies, Bowls & Treats: Easy Delicious Nutrition Recipes with Superfoods," we hope this culinary journey has been as enriching for you as it has been for us. This cookbook was crafted to provide recipes and guide you toward a path of wellness, one delicious and nutritious superfood-infused dish at a time.

This book's colorful array of recipes aims to inspire and tantalize your taste buds while nourishing your body with the powerful goodness of superfoods. From vibrant smoothie blends to hearty and nutrient-packed bowls and indulgent yet guilt-free treats, each recipe was designed to fit seamlessly into your lifestyle, balancing convenience and nourishment.

The vibrant full-color pictures adorning these pages were meant to accompany the recipes and motivate you to explore and replicate these creations in your kitchen. We believe that eating healthy doesn't mean sacrificing taste, and these visuals were carefully selected to reflect the vibrancy and deliciousness of the dishes.

We would love to hear about your journey through this cookbook. Your feedback is valuable to us and those just embarking on their wellness expedition. Your reviews, comments, and personal experiences with the recipes will serve as a guiding light for others who are seeking to embark on a similar path to healthier eating.

We invite you to share your thoughts, suggestions, and experiences while preparing these delightful dishes. Please leave your reviews on our website and share your thoughts on social media or with friends and family. Your input will help us improve and inspire others to embark on their culinary adventure.

Thank you for exploring the world of healthy smoothies, nourishing bowls, and guilt-free treats with us. We hope this book becomes your companion on your journey to a more wholesome and fulfilling lifestyle.

Wishing you vibrant health and culinary joy,

Emma Willson

SCAN ME

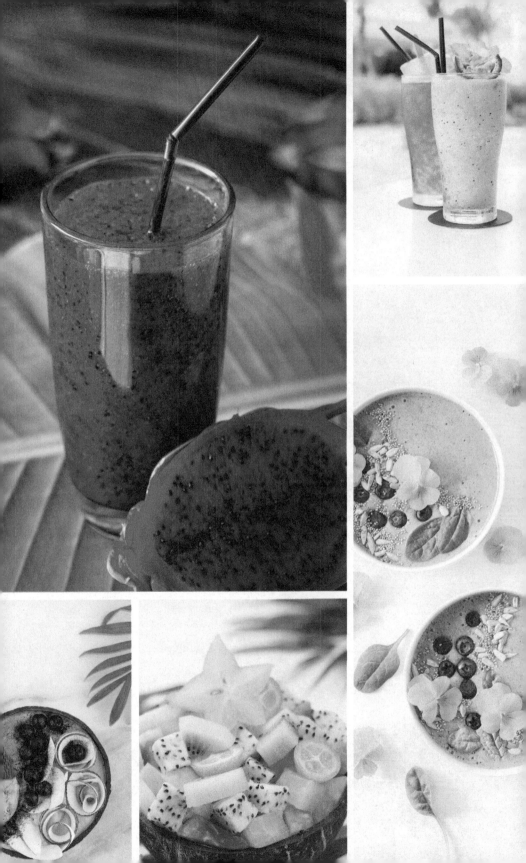

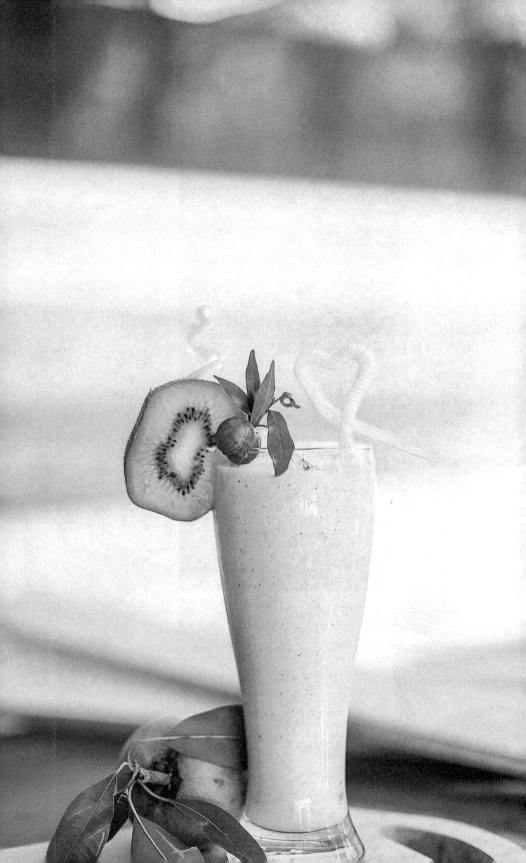

Made in the USA
Las Vegas, NV
19 December 2023

83186576R10046